How To Fix Damaged Hair Manual

A Step By Step Guide To Reverting Color, Heat and Protein Damage

AUTHOR BREANNA RUTTER

TABLE OF CONTENTS

INTRODUCTION TO
HOW TO FIX DAMAGED HAIR
MANUAL

"The How To Fix Damaged Hair Manual is a pocket guide that will help you to gain your healthy hair back since experiencing hair damage with your hair. There are a variety of reasons why you are experiencing damaged hair and the most common forms of hair damage that will be discussed in this manual is; heat damage, color damage, and protein damage. Growing your hair back to its most healthy state is a process that can be done in a variety of ways ranging from deep conditioning, protein treatments, daily moisturization, trimming damage split ends, Choosing healthy damage free hairstyling options, and so much more! Understanding how to care for your hair not only relies on your ability to diagnose what caused damage to your hair but also, how to treat it on a PH level!

Learning how to overcome damaged hair will take little hairstyling skills on your behalf because the solution to various hair damage issues are the treatments necessary for reversing their conditions. This manual will thoroughly educate you about understanding the prevention of hair damage from color, protein, and heat while suggesting hair care treatments that aid you in reversing its effects!

Please enjoy this informative read as you learn how to recover from damaged hair!"

-Sincerely Breanna

1 UNDERSTANDING HAIR PH

Have you experienced difficulty maintaining smooth frizz free hair? This is due part in large to keeping your hair PH balanced! Frizzy hair or damaged hair can ruin the look of many hairstyles with the most common being straight hair, twists, and braids. The reason why frizzy or damaged hair can be hard to beat is because the hair is not PH balanced! PH balance has a lot to do with the health and behavior of your hair especially when achieving certain looks. Your hair is left prone to breakage if it is not in its ideal range of PH!

The PH scale is used to measure how acidic or alkaline a solution is and the scale ranges from 1 (acidic) to 14 (alkaline). Water has a PH of 7 (neutral) and is used to compare the acidity or alkalinity of a solution. The ideal PH range of hair is 4.5 to 5.5. Hair has an acidity of 4.5 to 5.5 and should remain this way especially if you want to achieve your most healthy hair. The reason why this is important when reversing damaged hair is because when your hair is in contact with an acidic product, it will cause your cuticles (refer to definition guide) to flatten resulting in smooth & healthy moisturized strands of hair. When hair is in contact with an alkaline solution, the cuticles raise, the strands themselves swell (which can cause breakage) and results in frizzy, dry and ultimately, damaged hair!

When caring for your damaged hair, it is high priority to always keep your hair in the range of 4.5 to 5.5 and the best way to do this, is to make sure that you are using hair care products that are PH balanced. If you do not know the PH of your hair products, test your products with Litmus Strips. If you want products that are already PH balanced, I suggest HowToBlackHair.com referred hair care products specifically formulated for maintaining healthy hair.

2 UNDERSTANDING HAIR ELASTICITY

Have you ever experienced very stiff hair that lacks flow or movement while also breaking off easily? What about hair that is so limp and stretchy that it does not seem to hold a curl no matter what you do? The health of your hair not only relies on using PH balanced hair care products (between 4.5 to 5.5 acidity) but has everything to do with balancing the elasticity of your hair as well!

Incredibly stiff and sometimes brittle hair is the description for hair that has too much protein. Deep conditioning products is what this hair requires to have a healthy balance of elasticity. Not understanding how protein works on the hair has left many individuals to believe that they have protein sensitive hair and need to deep condition their hair more than once a week when this is never the case. Firstly, hair cannot be protein sensitive because it is actually made up of protein (keratin)! That statement is like saying you are allergic to water when our bodies are about 50-70% water! Instead of believing that your hair is protein sensitive, it's appropriate that you're just not in need of protein because for example, if you have relaxed hair, protein treatments are needed to prevent your hair from becoming weak and limp!

Weak and limp is exactly what describes hair that has a lack of protein. Protein products is what this hair requires to have a healthy balance of elasticity. A easy way to know if this hair needs protein is when it feels somewhat sticky when wet and if it is limp when wet or dry, especially when trying to hold curls. Protein will also benefit fine hair (refer to definition guide) greatly since fine hair can naturally feel limp and weaker than course hair (refer to definition guide).

3 COLOR DAMAGE+ TREATMENTS

Coloring your hair whether you have natural, relaxed, or transitioning can be done successfully without damage but damage is still a risk and many have unfortunately fell victim to color damage. Understanding why color damage happens and how it can be reverted relies partially on your understanding of the PH of hair.

Hair of course is in its most healthy state when it is maintained between an acidic PH of 4.5 to 5.5 and coloring your hair compromises that PH. Hair color is an alkaline product (higher than the PH of water) and because of this, it's state of PH raises the cuticles (refer to definition guide) and can cause the hair to swell double its size! This allows for the product to penetrate the cortex, where your hair color is stored, and either deposits (adds) or lifts (take away) color from your hair. Hair color varies in many forms and in order of most damaging to least damaging, color goes as followed; Bleaching, Permanent, Semi/Demi Permanent, and Plant Colorants. For more information on color, refer to The Relaxed Hair Bible to learn how color affects your hair as well as relaxed hair specifically.

Treating color damaged hair does not mean that you have to re-color your hair back to your original hair color, you have to incorporate shaft penetrating leave in protein and moisturizing products to maintain its ideal PH and elasticity. On the following page, you will be equipped with a treatment that allows you to repair your color damage and bring back your hair to its most healthy conditions!

If you are in need of quality PH balanced moisturizing and protein hair products, I highly suggest HowToBlackHair.com referred hair care products specifically formulated for maintaining healthy hair.

COLOR DAMAGE TREATMENT REGIMEN

DO NOT COLOR HAIR AGAIN UNTIL HAIR HAS
BECOME HEALTHY!

WEEK 1 DAY 1
Shampoo Wash (mandatory)
Deep Condition (mandatory)

WEEK 1 DAY 2
Protein Leave In (optional)

WEEK 1 DAY 3
Leave In Moisturizer (mandatory)

WEEK 1 DAY 4
Protein Leave In (optional)

WEEK 1 DAY 5
Leave In Moisturizer (mandatory)

WEEK 1 DAY 6
Protein Leave In (optional)

WEEK 1 DAY 7
Leave In Moisturizer (mandatory)

REPEAT REGIMEN WEEKLY UNTIL HAIR
BECOMES HEALTHY

REPLACE PROTEIN LEAVE IN WITH LEAVE IN
MOISTURIZER IF NEEDED!

4 HEAT DAMAGE + TREATMENTS

Those who suffer from heat damage can clearly see its effects especially if they have an existing pattern of hair whether it is curly, coily, or wavy. Heat damage prevents your natural pattern from reverting back to its natural state causing it to become limp and lifeless. Using heat, especially on already damaged hair, is extremely dangerous towards preserving the health of your hairs! Heat should only be used rarely, even on healthy hair, because heat causes a lot of problems, specifically when heat styling your hair. The only time heat usage is appropriate is if you are doing a Deep Conditioning or Protein Treatment because heat allows your cuticles to raise thus, allow the power of your treatment to produce intense results. When using heat for a hair treatment, heat is used all over your hair to encourage your products to penetrate your hair which is actually good for the health of it. If the heat is focused on your hair for heat styling, this can cause your hair to become weakened which results in thinning, breakage, and ultimately heat damage!

If you must use heat to style your hair, you have to test which setting is best for you and always use a heat protectant. Your preferred heat setting of choice should be the lowest setting on your styling tool that allows you to achieve your straightest result. For some, especially with fine or thin hair, their heat setting usually falls somewhere between 300° and 320° degrees. For those usually with thick or coarse hair, their heat setting will usually fall between 320° to 350°

Reverting from heat damage is not always successful and in most cases, trimming is required so refrain from using heat styling tools especially as you nurse your hair back to health!

HEAT DAMAGE TREATMENT REGIMEN

DO NOT HEAT STYLE AGAIN UNTIL HAIR HAS BECOME HEALTHY!

FOR HARD BRITTLE HAIR	FOR WEAK LIMP HAIR
WEEK 1 DAY 1 Shampoo Wash (mandatory) Deep Condition (mandatory)	WEEK 1 DAY 1 Shampoo Wash (mandatory) Protein Treatment (mandatory)
WEEK 1 DAY 2	WEEK 1 DAY 2
WEEK 1 DAY 3 Leave In Moisturizer (mandatory)	WEEK 1 DAY 3 Protein Leave In (mandatory)
WEEK 1 DAY 4	WEEK 1 DAY 4
WEEK 1 DAY 5 Leave In Moisturizer (mandatory)	WEEK 1 DAY 5 Protein Leave In (mandatory)
WEEK 1 DAY 6	WEEK 1 DAY 6
WEEK 1 DAY 7 Leave In Moisturizer (mandatory)	WEEK 1 DAY 7 Protein Leave In (mandatory)

REPEAT A GIVEN REGIMEN WEEKLY UNTIL HAIR BECOMES HEALTHY

INCREASE PROTEIN LEAVE IN OR LEAVE IN MOISTURIZER IF NEEDED!

TRIM DAMAGE IF HAIR DOES NOT REVERT AFTER 2 WEEK REGIMEN!

5 PROTEIN DAMAGE + TREATMENTS

Protein damaged hair requires deep condition treatments to release protein buildup from your hair and thankfully, protein damage (protein buildup) is reversible and I will explain to you how this is possible! The visible hair seen on your head is dead because its cells are no longer alive so hair is like a shell filled with your natural hair color with the ability to temporarily store added protein and moisture (water). That's why when you keep your hair dry for extended periods of time and use chemicals that compromises the health of your hair, this leaves your hair void of protein and moisture, which in unison, is needed to balance the elasticity of your hair.

Using a deep conditioner product will need to be performed frequently because if your hair is kept in this state of health, it will eventually begin to break and become increasingly damaged. A good guide for knowing how often to deep condition hair overloaded with protein, is at least every week or twice a week. How well your hair can bounce back with the help of deep conditioning will vary depending on your own unique head of hair. Also when deep conditioning your hair, remember to avoid adding product to your scalp as this will can cause buildup and create an irritable scalp!

On the following page, I will provide a deep conditioning regimen that should be performed weekly to release excessive protein from your hair. If you are in need of a quality deep conditioner for your hair, I highly suggest HowToBlackHair.com referred hair care products specifically formulated for maintaining healthy hair.

PROTEIN DAMAGE TREATMENT REGIMEN

DO NOT USE PRODUCTS
CONTAINING PROTEIN!

WEEK 1 DAY 1
Shampoo Wash (mandatory)
Deep Condition (mandatory)

WEEK 1 DAY 2
Leave In Moisturizer (mandatory)

WEEK 1 DAY 3
Leave In Moisturizer (mandatory)

WEEK 1 DAY 4
Leave In Moisturizer (mandatory)

WEEK 1 DAY 5
Leave In Moisturizer (mandatory)

WEEK 1 DAY 6
Leave In Moisturizer (mandatory)

WEEK 1 DAY 7
Leave In Moisturizer (mandatory)

REPEAT REGIMEN WEEKLY UNTIL HAIR
BECOMES HEALTHY

DECREASE LEAVE IN MOISTURIZER
IF NEEDED!

6 TRIMMING DAMAGED HAIR

Breakage is the aftermath of damaged hair so before damaged hair is encountered, it's important that you understand how to prevent damaged hair in the first place! The most popular forms of hair damage is usually from coloring, relaxing, heat styling, and rarely from an overload of protein. Implementing a Hair Care Regimen as well as incorporating Healthy Hair Care Habits, is the foundation for healthy flourishing hair. Its urgent that you have a specific regimen set in place to meet the hair care needs of your unique head of hair. Refer to the Natural Hair Bible, Relaxed Hair Bible, or Transitioning Hair Manual if you want to be thoroughly educated about how to care for your hair in its specific state of being.

Trimming damaged hair is a topic that has been heavily discussed in the various hair bibles and specific manuals because trimming is vital for reinforcing healthy hair and especially if you want to gain a longer length of hair. No matter if you keep your hair PH balanced or your Hair Elasticity is in check (which are both important), you will never see healthy ends if damaged ends aren't trimmed! Damaged ends will continue to break and split up the hair shaft (refer to definition guide) leaving you with short brittle hair if you do not step in and stop this condition from progressing!

On the following page, you will be provided with a Trimming Regimen that you can follow along with if you want to maintain healthy damage free hair as well as grow your hair to longer lengths. If you do not believe that you can successfully trim your damaged ends, please consult with a professional who can provide this service to you!

Transitioning Hair Trimming Relaxed Ends

ONLY USE CUTTING SHEARS EXCLUSIVELY USED FOR TRIMMING YOUR HAIR!

(TRIMMING DAMAGED ENDS W/ CURLY HAIR)

Step #1 Begin with damp detangled hair and position yourself in a well lit room with plenty of mirrors to help assist you

Step #2 Starting in the back of your head, part a horizontal line of hair at the nape of your neck and use gator clips/duck bill clips to keep the rest of your hair sectioned out of the way. Always work in small sections at a time!

Step #3 Take a small section of detangled hair, twist to the ends, and trim about an 1/8 inch of hair to dust for maintenance. Your dusted hair ends should look like little flecks of hair. For a trim that requires more than an 1/8 of length lost, consult with a professional to aid you so that you don't accidently give yourself an uneven trim.

(TRIMMING DAMAGED ENDS W/ STRAIGHT HAIR)

Step #1 Begin with dry detangled hair and position yourself in a well lit room with plenty of mirror to help assist you

Step #2 Follow Step 2 & Step 3 from above carefully

7 HEALTHY HAIRSTYLING OPTIONS

You must carefully consider your choice of hairstyling options and how much manipulation is required to complete a look you desire that can also preserve the health of your hair as well. Often times, hairstyling can be the culprit to many who have suffered with damaged hair but in this case, the suggested styles below will allow you to experience damage free styling! Below provided are lists of some of the worst and best hairstyles that encourage damaged hair and others that encourage damage free hair. One important thing to remember is that the more natural hairs you have contained within any given braid or twist, the stronger your hair will be in styles.

THE WORST HAIRSTYLES FOR DAMAGED HAIR
Micro Braids – small braids cause breakage easily
Kinky Twist (small) – small twists cause breakage easily
Ponytail Sew In – exposed hair can become heat damaged
Partial Sew In – exposed hair can become heat damaged
Quick Weave – glue can rip hair causing breakage
Heat Styling – can cause heat damage

THE BEST HAIRSTYLES FOR DAMAGED HAIR
Jumbo Individual Braids – large braids decrease breakage
Kinky Twists (large) – large twists decrease breakage
Net Weave Full Sew In – no hair exposed for heat damage
Invisible Part Sew In – concealed hair prevents heat damage
Roller Set – heat free coils
Flexi Rod Set – heat free curls
Straw Set – heat free coils
Bantu Knot Out – heat free waves/curls

There are many more choices that aren't listed here for

great hairstyles that can be worn on your hair so for more styling options, refer to HowToBlackHair.com

AFTERWORDS

"This manual was made in mind for those who desire step by step help with recovering from damaged hair whether it has been color damaged, heat damaged, or protein damaged! This manual offers a variety of solutions that will help you to resolve your issues because every single damage issue is unique to its own recovery needs. For example, hair that is overload with protein needs an intense amount of daily moisturization to "cancel out" in a way, the extra protein stored inside of your hair follicles. As you may have read throughout these chapters, implementing some simple but practical hair care solutions, is how you will be able to get on track to its most healthy state of being. You may have chosen to read this guide because you support my work, you were looking for information on recovering from damaged hair, or you were looking for this information to help a loved one.

Personally, I have never suffered from heat, color, or protein damage but I have had many close calls with them! What I have suffered greatly with was dry brittle hair! I have never shared with others my experience on coloring hair but in my book, The Relaxed Hair Bible, I discussed in detail the things I went through with my hair in my younger years, and why I decided to abandon coloring my hair. At that time, I was also relaxing my hair inappropriately which is also discussed there and through those experiences, I have learned firsthand my lessons on healthy hair care and how important a hair care foundation is. If you continue to practice good hair care and hairstyling habits, your hair will continue to flourish and remain healthy.

I hope that you thoroughly enjoyed this read, it was a pleasure of mine to write this for your knowledge and enjoyment." - Sincerely, Breanna

ADDITIONAL RESOURCES

The Official Website: www.Howtoblackhair.com

The Online Store: www.HowtoblackhairStore.com

Free Subscription Email: http://eepurl.com/FZs5b

For Additional Hair Questions

YourHairQuestions@Gmail.com

Black Hair Styling Tutorials

BlackWomenHair YouTube Channel

www.Youtube.com/BlackWomenHair

HowToBlackHair YouTube Channel

www.Youtube.com/HowToBlackHair

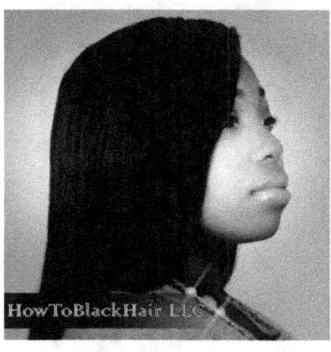

The Natural Hair Bible

The 10 Commandments of Black Hair Care

www.HowToBlackHair.com

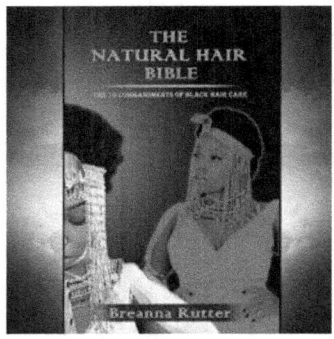

The Relaxed Hair Bible

The 10 Commandments of Long Healthy Relaxed Hair

www.HowToBlackHair.com

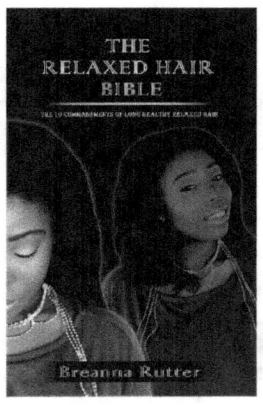

Black Hair Styling DVDs (Over 20+ Hairstyles)

www.HowToBlackHair.com

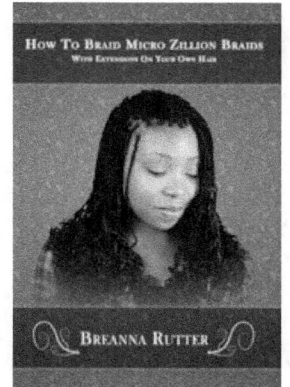 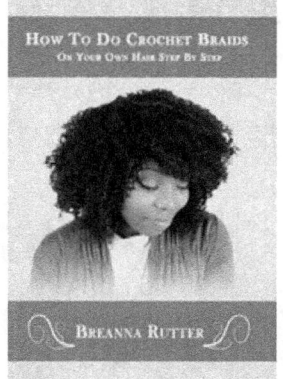

DEFINITION GUIDE

Cuticles: *a naturally protecting shield (arranged like shingles to the roof of a home) outside of your hair strands*

Cortex: *the innermost part of your hair follicle*

Course Hair: *your individual strands of hair are the same size or bigger in size (diameter) to regular sewing thread*

Elasticity: *the stretching ability of your hair*

Fine Hair: *your individual strands of hair are smaller in size (diameter) to regular sewing thread*

PH Balance: *hair balanced with a PH of 4.5 to 5.5*

Shaft: *the visibly seen strands of hair*

Thick Hair: *your ponytail width, with all of your hair gathered, is the width of a quarter or larger*

Thin Hair: *your ponytail width, with all of your hair gathered, is the width of a nickel or smaller*

INDEX

HOW TO BLACK HAIR LLC.
WRITTEN BY BREANNA RUTTER
BOOK DESIGNED BY BREANNA RUTTER
COVER DESIGNED BY JARED RUTTER
ALL RIGHTS RESERVED.
VISIT WWW.HOWTOBLACKHAIR.COM

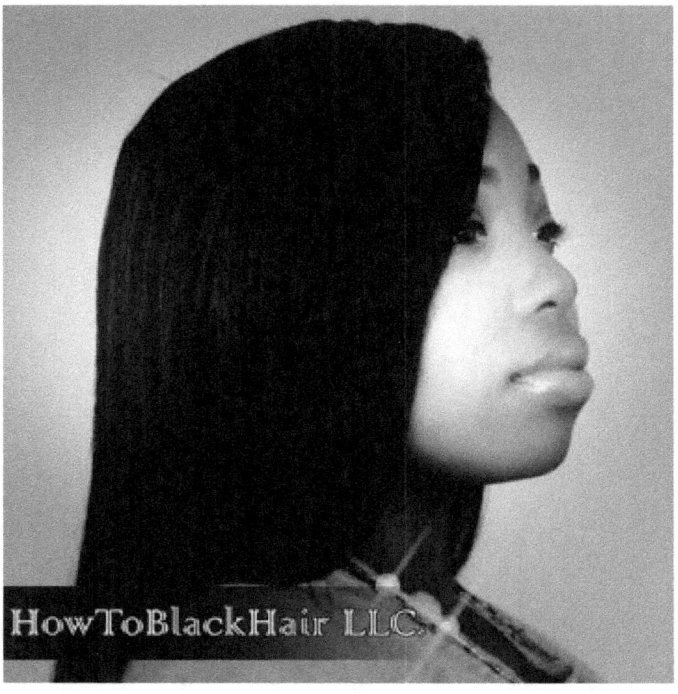